# PREFACE

OSCE or Objective Structured Clinical Examination is conducted by some specified universities in UK under guidance from Nurses and Midwifery Council (NMC). You can book your OSCE at any of the university website, provided you should have the decision letter from Nurses and Midwifery Council, UK. In simple words, OSCE is a practical exam in a simulated scenario. There will be only actors or Mannequins.

There is a total of 8 stations in NMC OSCE. This includes Assessment, Planning, Implementation, Evaluation stations (The APIE Stations), Evidence Based Practice, Professional Values and also the Skills (involves four) station.

This book might be of big help for those nurses who want practice OSCE with friends before attempting exam. This book is based on 'Adult OSCE Marking Criteria' laid down by mutual consensus of universities which are conducting OSCE.

**The APIE Stations**

**A - Assessment Station**

In assessment station you need to assess a patient (actor) or a mannequin within 15 minutes of commencing the exam. Assessment can be a neurological assessment, NEWS2 assessment (National Early Warning Scale 2) or a community assessment. You need to calculate the GCS score or NEWS2 score or PHQ9 score respectively in each station. This includes charting of vital signs in the given observation chart and explaining to the patient about the score attained along with plan of escalation of care. You also need to ask questions peculiar to the scenario. There are various assessment criteria as per university documents.

## P - Planning Station

After assessment station, next one is the Planning station in APIE Stations of NMC OSCE. Planning station is a silent station and time duration is another 14 minutes. In this station, you will be provided with the observation you charted in your assessment station and you need to write two care plans prioritizing the problems of the patient.

## I - Implementation Station

In implementation station of NMC OSCE, you will be provided a drug chart and you need to administer medication to a mannequin. In the given drug chart, details about weight, height, allergies, stat medications, prn medications and regular medications etc. will be prescribed. You need to read aloud the whole prescription, identify patient twice, make note of allergies and medications already administered and you need to administer the oral drugs due at that point of time. Time limit for implementation station is 15 minutes.

## E - Evaluation Station

In evaluation station has changed from previous module of OSCE. At present Evaluation station is a six-minute station in which you will get ready for an SBAR hand over of the patient. You will be provided with all the examination papers of API stations. This is not a silent station now.

## Professional Values and Behaviors

This is a silent writing osce station different from Legacy OSCE. Here, five topics are usually asked and you need to have a clear picture about marking criteria of each of them. Time limit is 10 minutes

## Evidence Based Practice (EBP) station

This is another new, silent writing station added to NMC OSCE. There is five topics to be learnt in this station. You need to make sure that you have learnt properly the marking criteria for each of those topics. Time limit is 10 minutes.

## Skills Station

You will need to demonstrate four skills during your NMC OSCE. All the skills have different time limits now. Sometimes you will be asked to perform two skills together as well. It can be any of the following,

Pressure Area Assessment

Pain Assessment

Midstream collection of urine and urinalysis

Fluid Balance Calculation

Fine bore NG insertion

Administration of Inhaled Medication

Aseptic Non-Touch Technique (ANTT)

IV flush and visual infusion phlebitis

Peak Flow Meter (PFM)

Basic Life Support (BLS)

Removal of Urinary Catheter

Catheter Urine Sample Collection

Injections

**From November 2022, following skills have been added to NMC OSCE**

- Administration of Suppository

- Bowel Assessment

- Nasopharyngeal Suctioning

- Nutritional assessment

- Oral Care Plan

- Oxygen therapy.

Evidence based practice station and Professional values station are silent stations only meant to write the interventions according to scenario. They are quite self-explanatory which candidates need to self-study. That's the reason we haven't included those two stations in this book.

We have included provision to give feedback to candidate after attempting each skill or station in OSCE. Feedback will be of three categories – Fully met, Partially Met or Not met (Scores 2, 1 and 0 respectively).

If you like to read step by step review of each station and skills please have a look on our previously published book – 'NMC OSCE for Overseas Nurses' by Lovelyn Joshi or go through free articles on our website which is https://www.oscetrainer.com. This book is mainly intended to guide you through trial-and-error practice of each station and skills.

Happy Learning and All the best for your OSCE.....Lovelyn Joshi

# Disclaimer

*Although the publisher and the author have made every effort to ensure that the information in this book was correct at press time and while this publication is designed to provide accurate information in regard to the subject matter covered, the publisher and the author assume no responsibility for errors, inaccuracies, omissions, or any other inconsistencies herein and hereby disclaim any liability to any party for any loss, damage, or disruption caused by errors or omissions, whether such errors or omissions result from negligence, accident, or any other cause.*

*PLEASE NOTE THAT MARKING CRITERIA IS THE ONLY DOCUMENT RELEASED BY UNIVERSITIES TO PRACTICE PERFECT FOR YOUR OSCE. ALL THE OTHER RECOMMENDATIONS AND SUGGESSTIONS MENTIONED IN THIS BOOK IS TO AID YOUR DECISION MAKING SKILL.*

# ASSESSMENT STATION

| Feedback Score: | Attempt: | 1 | 2 | 3 | 4 | 5 |
|---|---|---|---|---|---|---|
| Fully Met (2) Partially Met (1) Not Met (0) | Date & Name: | | | | | |
| 1 | Assesses the safety of the scene and the privacy and dignity of the patient. | | | | | |
| 2 | Cleans hands with alcohol hand rub, or washes with soap and water and dries with paper towels, following WHO guidelines. | | | | | |
| 3 | Introduces self to person. | | | | | |
| 4 | Check's identity with patient (the person's name is essential, and either their date of birth or hospital number) verbally, against wristband (where appropriate) and documentation. | | | | | |
| 5 | Checks for allergies verbally and on wrist band (where appropriate). | | | | | |
| 6 | Gains consent and explains reason for the assessment. | | | | | |
| 7 | Uses a calm voice, speech is clear, body language is open, personal space is appropriate. | | | | | |

| 8 | Airway: Clear; no visual obstructions. | | | | | | |
|---|---|---|---|---|---|---|---|
| 9 | Breathing: Respiratory rate; rhythm; depth; oxygen saturation level; respiratory noises (rattle wheeze, stridor, coughing); unequal air entry; visual signs of respiratory distress (use of accessory respiratory muscles, sweating, cyanosis, 'see-saw' breathing). | | | | | | |
| 10 | Circulation: Heart rate; rhythm; strength; blood pressure; capillary refill; pallor and perfusion. | | | | | | |
| 11 | Disability: conscious level using ACVPU (alert, confusion, voice, pain, unresponsive); presence of pain; urine output; blood glucose. | | | | | | |
| 12 | Exposure: Takes and records temperature; asks for the presence of bleeds, rashes, injuries and/ or bruises: obtains a medical history. | | | | | | |
| 13 | Accurately measures and documents the patient's vital signs and specific assessment tools. | | | | | | |
| 14 | Calculates National Early Warning Score (NEWS) or Glasgow coma scale accurately. | | | | | | |
| 15 | Accurately completes document: signs, adds date and time on assessment charts. | | | | | | |
| 16 | Conducts a holistic assessment relevant to the patient's scenario. | | | | | | |
| 17 | Disposes of equipment | | | | | | |

| | | | | | | | |
|---|---|---|---|---|---|---|---|
| | appropriately – verbalisation accepted. | | | | | | |
| 18 | Cleans hands with alcohol hand rub, or washes with soap and water and dries with paper towels, following WHO guidelines – verbalisation accepted. | | | | | | |
| 19 | Acts professionally throughout the procedure in accordance with NMC (2018) 'The Code: Professional standards of practice and behaviour for nurses, midwives and nursing associates". | | | | | | |

## **RED FLAGS**

If the candidate fails to acknowledge the actor and/or communicate effectively. For example, there is no or minimal eye contact, has their back to the patient, mumbles or has unclear verbal communications.

If the candidate is actively dismissive of the patient's complaint, concerns/anxieties.

If the candidate fails to accurately record physiological observations on the NEWS chart.

If the candidate fails to calculate the NEWS score accurately.

If the candidate fails to conduct an A – E assessment.

If the candidate fails to escalate concerning behaviour, or a deterioration in health (significant escalation in NEWS score)

If the candidate fails to escalate concerning behaviour, or a deterioration in health (significant escalation in NEWS score).

If the candidate fails to acknowledge or record the main care needs of the patient.

If the candidate openly displays judgemental behaviour about a patient's personal characteristics (e.g. sexuality), belief/cultural/lifestyle preferences.

If the candidate actively fails to utilise appropriate PPE causing risk to themselves and the patient.

If a candidate physically causes intentional harm to the patient through resistant and/ or unnecessary procedures.

Another red flag issue (leading directly to patient harm) identified by assessor.

# <u>Notes</u>

# PLANNING STATION

| Feedback Score: | Attempt: | 1 | 2 | 3 | 4 | 5 |
|---|---|---|---|---|---|---|
| **Fully Met (2)** **Partially Met (1)** **Not Met (0)** | **Date & Name:** | | | | | |
| 1 | Clearly and legibly handwrites answers. | | | | | |
| 2 | Identifies two relevant nursing problems/needs. | | | | | |
| 3 | Sets appropriate evaluation date for both problems. | | | | | |
| 4 | Ensures nursing interventions are current/evidence based/best practice. | | | | | |
| 5 | Uses professional terminology in care planning. | | | | | |
| 6 | Does not use abbreviations or acronyms. | | | | | |
| 7 | Ensures strike through errors retain legibility. | | | | | |
| 8 | Accurately prints, signs and dates. | | | | | |
| 9 | Act professionally throughout the procedure in accordance with NMC (2016) 'The Code: Professional standards of practice and behaviour for | | | | | |

| | nurses, midwives and nursing associates' | | | | | | |
|---|---|---|---|---|---|---|---|

## RED FLAGS

If the candidates fail to acknowledge or record the main care needs of the patient

If the candidate openly displays judgemental behaviour about a patient's personal characteristics (e.g. Sexuality), belief/cultural/ lifestyle preferences.

Another red flag issue (leading directly to patient harm) identified by assessor.

# **Notes**

# IMPLEMENTATION STATION

| Feedback Score: | Attempt: | 1 | 2 | 3 | 4 | 5 |
|---|---|---|---|---|---|---|
| Fully Met (2) Partially Met (1) Not Met (0) | Date & Name: | | | | | |
| 1 | Cleans hands with alcohol hand rub, or washes with soap and water and dries with paper towels, following who guidelines. | | | | | |
| 2 | Introduces self to the person. | | | | | |
| 3 | Seeks consent from the person or carer prior to administering medication. | | | | | |
| 4 | Checks allergies on chart and confirms with the person in their care; also notes red ID wristband (where appropriate). | | | | | |
| 5 | Before administering any prescribed drug, looks at person's prescription chart and correctly checks all the following: Correct: Person (checks id with person: verbally, against wrist band (where appropriate) and documentation)-drug-dose- | | | | | |

| | | | | | | |
|---|---|---|---|---|---|---|
| | date and time of administration-route and method of administration-diluent (as appropriate). | | | | | |
| 6 | Correctly checks all the following-Validity of prescription-Signature of prescriber - Prescription is legible. If any of these pieces of information is missing, unclear or illegible, the nurse should not proceed with administration and should consult the prescriber. | | | | | |
| 7 | Considers contraindication where relevant and medical information prior to administration (prompt permitted). (This may not be relevant in all scenarios). | | | | | |
| 8 | Provides a correct explanation of what each drug being administered is for the person in their care (Prompt permitted). | | | | | |
| 9 | Administers drugs due for administration correctly and safely. | | | | | |
| 10 | Omits drugs not to be administered and provides verbal rationale. (Ask the candidate the reason for non-administration if not verbalised). | | | | | |
| 11 | Accurately documents drug administration and non-administration, including the details of the person administering the medication. | | | | | |
| 12 | Act professionally throughout the procedure in accordance | | | | | |

| | with NMC (2016) 'The Code: Professional standards of practice and behaviour for nurses, midwives and nursing associates. | | | | | |
|---|---|---|---|---|---|---|

## RED FLAGS

If the candidate fails to acknowledge the actor and/or communicate effectively. For example: there is no or minimal eye contact, has their back to the patient, mumbles or has unclear verbal communications.

If the candidate ignores or fails to check allergy status and risks causing a reaction prior to the administration of medicine.

If the candidate makes a drug error during the administration of medication.

If the candidate fails to accurately sign and date the drug chart.

If the candidate openly displays judgemental behaviour about a patient's personal characteristics (e.g., sexuality), belief/cultural/ lifestyle preferences.

If the candidate actively fails to utilise appropriate PPE causing risk to themselves and the patient.

If a candidate physically causes intentional harm to the patient through restraint and or unnecessary procedures.

Another Red flag issue (leading directly to patient harm) identified by assessor.

# **<u>Notes</u>**

# EVALUATION STATION

| Feedback Score: | Attempt: | 1 | 2 | 3 | 4 | 5 |
|---|---|---|---|---|---|---|
| Fully Met (2) Partially Met (1) Not Met (0) | Date & Name: | | | | | |
| 1 | **Situation** | | | | | |
| 1A | Introduces self and the clinical setting. | | | | | |
| 1B | States the patient's name, hospital number and or date of birth and location. | | | | | |
| 1C | States the reason for the handover (where relevant). | | | | | |
| 2 | **Background** | | | | | |
| 2A | States date of admission/visit/ reason for initial admission/ referral to specialist team and diagnosis. | | | | | |
| 2B | Notes previous medical history and relevant medication/social history/allergies. | | | | | |
| 2C | Gives details of current events and details the findings from assessment. | | | | | |
| 3 | **Assessment** | | | | | |

| | | | | | | | |
|---|---|---|---|---|---|---|---|
| 3A | States most recent observations, any results from assessments undertaken and what changes have occurred. | | | | | | |
| 3B | Identifies main nursing needs. | | | | | | |
| 3C | States nursing and medical interventions completed (care plan/drug chart). | | | | | | |
| 3D | States areas of concerns (Evaluation scenario). | | | | | | |
| 4 | **Recommendation** | | | | | | |
| 4A | States what is required of the person taking the handover and proposes a realistic plan of action. | | | | | | |
| 5 | Verbal communication is clear and appropriate. | | | | | | |
| 6 | Systematic and structured approach taken to handover. | | | | | | |
| 7 | Act professionally throughout the procedure in accordance with NMC (2016) 'The Code: Professional standards of practice and behaviour for nurses, midwives and nursing associates. | | | | | | |

## RED FLAGS

If the candidate fails to acknowledge or record the main care needs of the patient.

If the candidate openly displays judgemental behaviour about a patient's personal characteristics (e.g., Sexuality), belief/cultural/ lifestyle preferences.

If a candidate fails to clearly and accurately communicate with the healthcare professional when handing care of the patient over.

Another Red Flag Issue (leading directly to patient harm) identified by assessor.

# **Notes**

# SKILLS

# WOUND ASSESSMENT

| Feedback Score: | Attempt: | 1 | 2 | 3 | 4 | 5 |
|---|---|---|---|---|---|---|
| **Fully Met (2) Partially Met (1) Not Met (0)** | **Date & Name:** | | | | | |
| 1 | Checks that the patient is comfortable and verbalises that a pain assessment will be undertaken prior to procedure. | | | | | |
| 2 | Cleans hands with alcohol hand rub, or washes with soap and water and dries with paper towels. | | | | | |
| 3 | Dons a disposable plastic apron and non-sterile gloves. | | | | | |
| 4 | Assesses and reports the condition of the wound: Examines for erythema Describes the area around the wound Describes any exudate (pus, bleed) Describes the defect in the closure Describes the condition of the floor of the defect | | | | | |

| | | | | | | | |
|---|---|---|---|---|---|---|---|
| | Asks about pain and tenderness. | | | | | | |
| 5 | Disposes of waste appropriately - verbalisation accepted. | | | | | | |
| 6 | Describes any further actions that should be taken, such as swab and referral to the medical team. | | | | | | |

## RED FLAGS

Any Red Flag Issue (leading directly to patient harm) identified by assessor.

# <u>**Notes**</u>

# ASEPTIC NON-TOUCH TECHNIQUE (ANTT)

| Feedback Score: | Attempt: | 1 | 2 | 3 | 4 | 5 |
|---|---|---|---|---|---|---|
| **Fully Met (2)** **Partially Met (1)** **Not Met (0)** | **Date & Name:** | | | | | |
| 1 | Cleans hands with alcohol hand rub and dons' disposable gloves and apron. | | | | | |
| 2 | Cleans trolley with detergent wipes (or equivalent) from further to nearest point. | | | | | |
| 3 | Removes and disposes of gloves and apron. Cleans hands with alcohol hand rub. | | | | | |
| 4 | Checks that all the equipment required for the procedure is available and, where applicable, is sterile (i.e., that packaging is undamaged, intact and dry, and that sterility indicators are present on any sterilised items and have changed colour where applicable). | | | | | |
| 5 | Places all the equipment required for the procedure on | | | | | |

| | | | | | | |
|---|---|---|---|---|---|---|
| | the bottom shelf of the clean dressing trolley (or suitable equivalent). (Equipment: sterile dressing pack, Nail 0.9% for cleaning, alcohol cleaning wipes, wound dressing, alcohol hand rub, disposable apron). | | | | | |
| 6 | Takes the trolley to the person's bedside, disturbing the curtains as little as possible. | | | | | |
| 7 | Cleans hands with alcohol hand rub, or washes with soap and water, dries with paper towels, following WHO guidelines. | | | | | |
| 8 | Dons a disposable plastic apron. | | | | | |
| 9 | Opens the outer cover of the sterile pack and, having verified that the pack is the correct way up, slides the contents, without touching them, onto the top shelf of the trolley (or suitable equivalent). | | | | | |
| 10 | Cleans hands with alcohol hand rub. | | | | | |
| 11 | Opens the sterile field using only the corners of the paper. | | | | | |
| 12 | Opens any other packs, tipping their contents gently onto the centre of the sterile field. Uses alcohol wipe to clean the saline solution for 30 seconds, allowing it to dry for 30 seconds. | | | | | |
| 13 | Cleans hands with alcohol hand rub and dons' sterile gloves. | | | | | |
| 14 | Carries out and completes the relevant procedure using ANTT: | | | | | |

| | | | | | | |
|---|---|---|---|---|---|---|
| | Drapes sterile field around/ under the wound area. States which hand will be 'clean' and which will be 'dirty' Dips gauze in saline solution, moving from the clean to dirty hand. Cleans wound from clean to dirty areas in a single stroke, taking care not to over clean the wound. Applies new dressing. Avoids contaminating sterile field or the key parts at all times. | | | | | |
| 15 | Replaces bedcovers. | | | | | |
| 16 | Disposes of waste appropriately - verbalisation accepted. | | | | | |
| 17 | Cleans hands with alcohol hand rub, or washes with soap and water and dries with paper towels, following WHO guidelines - Verbalisation accepted. | | | | | |
| 18 | Checks the person is comfortable and is able to reach the call buzzer. | | | | | |
| 19 | Act professionally throughout the procedure in accordance with NMC (2016) 'The Code: Professional standards of practice and behaviour for nurses, midwives and nursing associates'. | | | | | |

## RED FLAGS

Candidate who obviously contaminate the sterile field or are unable to recognise the sterile field (If contaminated, immediate rectification or verbalisation of error to the examiner is needed).

Another Red Flag issue (leading directly to patient harm)

identified by assessor.

# <u>Notes</u>

# INTRAMUSCULAR INJECTION

| Feedback Score: | Attempt: | 1 | 2 | 3 | 4 | 5 |
|---|---|---|---|---|---|---|
| Fully Met (2) Partially Met (1) Not Met (0) | Date & Name: | | | | | |
| 1 | Explains and discusses the procedure with the person. | | | | | |
| 2 | Before administering any prescribed drug, looks at the person's prescription chart and correctly checks all of the following: Correct person (checks id with person: verbally, against wristband (where appropriate and documentation), drug, dos, date and time of administration, route and method of administration, diluent (as appropriate)-any allergies. | | | | | |
| 3 | Correctly checks all of the following:<br>- Validity of prescription.<br>- Signature of prescriber.<br>- Prescription is legible. | | | | | |

| | | | | | | |
|---|---|---|---|---|---|---|
| | If any of these pieces of information is missing, unclear or illegible, the nurse should not proceed with administration and should consult the prescriber. | | | | | |
| 4 | Cleans hands with alcohol hand rub, or washes with soap and water and dries with paper towels, following WHO guidelines. | | | | | |
| 5 | Assembles equipment required and prepares medication. | | | | | |
| 6 | Dons a disposable plastic apron. Closes the curtains/door and assists the person into the required position. Removes the appropriate garment to expose injection site. | | | | | |
| 7 | Assesses the injection site for signs of inflammation, oedema, infection and skin lesions. | | | | | |
| 8 | Cleans hands with alcohol hand rub, or washes with soap and water and dries with paper towels, following WHO guidelines. Dons non sterile gloves. | | | | | |
| 9 | Cleans injection site with a swab saturated with isopropyl alcohol 70% for 30 seconds and allows to dry for 30 seconds. | | | | | |
| 10 | Stretches the skin around the injection site. | | | | | |
| 11 | Inserts the needle at an angle of 90 degree into the skin until about 1cm of the needle is left showing. | | | | | |

| 12 | Depresses the plunger at approximately 1ml every 10 seconds and injects the drug slowly. (Only if using dorso-gluteal muscles: pulls back on the plunger to check for blood aspiration) | | | | | | |
|----|----|---|---|---|---|---|---|
| 13 | Waits 10 seconds before withdrawing the needle. | | | | | | |
| 14 | Withdraws the needle rapidly. Applies gentle pressure to any bleeding point but does not massage the site. | | | | | | |
| 15 | Applies a small plaster over the puncture site. | | | | | | |
| 16 | Ensures that all sharps and non - sharp waste are disposed of safely (including scooping method of re - sheathing and transportation of sharps) and in accordance with locally approved procedures. | | | | | | |
| 17 | Cleans hands with alcohol hand rub, or washes with soap and water and dries with paper towels, following WHO guidelines - Verbalisation accepted. | | | | | | |
| 18 | Dates and signs drug documentation (prompt permitted) | | | | | | |
| 19 | Act professionally throughout the procedure in accordance with NMC (2016) 'The Code: Professional standards of practice and behaviour for nurses, midwives and nursing associates' | | | | | | |

## RED FLAGS

Safety of administration of medication. This should include checking the prescription against the patient, and checking right dose/right time/right patient/right route/right drug. The chart should be timed and signed. If any of the above is missed, this should result in a fail for this station.

Another Red Flag issue (leading directly to patient harm) identified by assessor.

# <u>Notes</u>

# SUBCUTANEOUS INJECTION

| Feedback Score: | Attempt: | 1 | 2 | 3 | 4 | 5 |
|---|---|---|---|---|---|---|
| **Fully Met (2) Partially Met (1) Not Met (0)** | **Date & Name:** | | | | | |
| 1 | Explains and discusses the procedure with the person. | | | | | |
| 2 | Before administering any prescribed drug, looks at the person's prescription chart and correctly checks all of the following: Correct person (checks id with person: verbally, against wristband (where appropriate and documentation), drug, dos, date and time of administration, route and method of administration, diluent (as appropriate)-any allergies. | | | | | |
| 3 | Correctly checks all of the following:<br>- Validity of prescription.<br>- Signature of prescriber.<br>- Prescription is legible. | | | | | |

| | | | | | | |
|---|---|---|---|---|---|---|
| | If any of these pieces of information is missing, unclear or illegible, the nurse should not proceed with administration and should consult the prescriber. | | | | | |
| 4 | Cleans hands with alcohol hand rub, or washes with soap and water and dries with paper towels following WHO guidelines. Dons a disposable plastic apron. | | | | | |
| 5 | Assembles equipment required and prepares medication using non touch technique. | | | | | |
| 6 | Closes the curtains/door and assists the person into the required position. Removes the appropriate garment to expose injection site. | | | | | |
| 7 | Assesses the injection site for signs of inflammation, oedema, infection and skin lesions. Rotates injection sites if having regular injections. | | | | | |
| 8 | Cleans hands with alcohol hand rub, or washes with soap and water and dries with paper towels. Dons non - sterile gloves. | | | | | |
| 9 | States would assess the cleanliness of the injection site. States that if the site is clean there would be no need to clean, however if required would clean with a swab saturated with isopropyl alcohol 70% for 30 seconds and allows to dry for 30 | | | | | |

| | | | | | | | |
|---|---|---|---|---|---|---|---|
| | seconds. | | | | | | |
| 10 | Removes the needle sheath. | | | | | | |
| 11 | Gently pinches the skin into a fold. | | | | | | |
| 12 | Holds the needle between thumb and forefinger of dominant hand as if grasping a dart. | | | | | | |
| 13 | Inserts the needle into the skin at an angle of 90 degrees (necessary for administration of insulin) and releases the grasped skin. (An angle of 45 degree is permitted if the candidate considers the person to have less subcutaneous tissue present or if administering medication other than insulin.) | | | | | | |
| 14 | Injects the medicine slowly over 10 to 30 seconds. | | | | | | |
| 15 | Withdraws the needle rapidly and applies gentle pressure with sterile gauze. Does not massage the area. | | | | | | |
| 16 | Ensures that all sharps and non - sharp waste are disposed of safely (including scooping method of re - sheathing and transportation of sharps) and in accordance with locally approved procedures. | | | | | | |
| 17 | Cleans hands with alcohol hand rub, or washes with soap and water and dries with paper towels, following WHO guidelines - verbalisation accepted. | | | | | | |

| 18 | Signs and dates medicines administration record (prompt permitted). | | | | | |
|----|----|---|---|---|---|---|
| 19 | Act professionally throughout the procedure in accordance with NMC (2016) 'The Code: Professional standards of practice and behaviour for nurses, midwives and nursing associates' | | | | | |

## RED FLAGS

Safety of administration of medication

Administration should include the following essential criteria:

Right patient/right route/right drug/right time/right dose.

The drug chart should be signed, timed and dated.

If any of the above is missed, it should result in a n automatic fail.

Incorrect injection technique. Either failure to deliver at 45-degree angle or not pinching the skill

# <u>Notes</u>

# REMOVAL OF URINARY CATHETER

| Feedback Score: | Attempt: | 1 | 2 | 3 | 4 | 5 |
|---|---|---|---|---|---|---|
| **Fully Met (2)** **Partially Met (1)** **Not Met (0)** | **Date & Name:** | | | | | |
| 1 | Explains the procedure to the person and informs them of potential post catheter symptoms such as urgency, frequency and discomfort, which are often caused by irritation of the urethra by the catheter. | | | | | |
| 2 | Assembles the equipment required. | | | | | |
| 3 | Cleans hands with alcohol hand rub, or washes with soap and water and dries with paper towels, following WHO guidelines. | | | | | |
| 4 | Dons a disposable plastic apron and non-sterile gloves. | | | | | |
| 5 | Having checked volume of water in balloon (see patient documentation), uses syringe to | | | | | |

| | | | | | | | |
|---|---|---|---|---|---|---|---|
| | deflate balloon in full. | | | | | | |
| 6 | Asks person to breathe in and then out. As person exhales, gently but firmly with continuous traction removes catheter. | | | | | | |
| 7 | Cleans and dries area around the genitalia and makes the person comfortable. | | | | | | |
| 8 | Encourages person to exercised and to drink 2.5 litres of fluids per day. | | | | | | |
| 9 | Disposes of equipment including apron and gloves appropriately - verbalisation accepted. | | | | | | |
| 10 | Cleans hands with alcohol hand rub, or washes with soap and water and dries with paper towels following WHO guidelines - verbalisation accepted. | | | | | | |
| 11 | Verbalises asking the patient to inform the nurse when urine has been passed. | | | | | | |
| 12 | Act professionally throughout the procedure in accordance with NMC (2016) 'The Code: Professional standards of practice and behaviour for nurses, midwives and nursing associates'. | | | | | | |

## RED FLAGS

If the candidate does not deflate the balloon prior to removal, this should result in a fail for this station.

Another Red flag issue (leading directly to patient harm) identified by assessor.

# <u>Notes</u>

# CATHETER SPECIMEN OF URINE (CSU)

| Feedback Score: | Attempt: | 1 | 2 | 3 | 4 | 5 |
|---|---|---|---|---|---|---|
| **Fully Met (2) Partially Met (1) Not Met (0)** | **Date & Name:** | | | | | |
| 1 | Explains and discusses the procedure with the person. | | | | | |
| 2 | Checks that any equipment required for the procedure is available and, where applicable, is sterile (i.e. that packaging is undamaged, intact and dry, is within the expiration date, that sterility indicators are present on any sterilised items and have changed colour, where applicable). | | | | | |
| 3 | If no urine is visible in the catheter tubing: cleans hands with alcohol hand rub, or washes with soap and water and dries with paper towels, dons a disposable plastic apron and non-sterile gloves prior to manipulating the catheter tubing. | | | | | |

| | | | | | | |
|---|---|---|---|---|---|---|
| 4 | Applies non-traumatic clamp a few centimetres distal to the sampling port. Removes gloves and disposes appropriately. | | | | | |
| 5 | Cleans hands with alcohol hand rub, or washes with soap and water and dries with paper towels, following WHO guidelines. | | | | | |
| 6 | Dons non sterile gloves. | | | | | |
| 7 | Wipes sampling port with 2% chlorhexidine in 70% isopropyl alcohol and allows tying for 30 seconds. | | | | | |
| 8 | If using needle and syringe: Inserts needle into port at an angle of 45 degree, using a non-touch technique, and aspirates the required amount of urine, then withdraws needle. If using needless system: Inserts sterile syringe firmly into centre of sampling port (according to manufacturer's guidelines) using a non-touch technique, aspirates the required amount of urine, and removes syringe. | | | | | |
| 9 | Transfers an adequate volume of the urine specimen (approximately 10 ml) into a sterile container immediately. | | | | | |
| 10 | Discards needle and syringe into sharps container (if relevant). | | | | | |
| 11 | Wipes sampling port with 2% chlorhexidine in 70% isopropyl alcohol and allows drying for 30 seconds. | | | | | |

| 12 | Unclamps catheter tubing (if relevant). | | | | | |
| 13 | Disposes of equipment including apron and gloves appropriately - verbalisation accepted. | | | | | |
| 14 | Cleans hands with alcohol hand rub, or washes with soap and water and dries with paper towels, following WHO guidelines - verbalisation accepted. | | | | | |
| 15 | Verbalises the need to label the container correctly and place into microbiology bag ready to send to laboratory as soon as the sample is obtained. | | | | | |
| 16 | Acts professionally throughout the procedure in accordance with NMC (2018) 'The Code: Professional standards of practice and behaviour for nurses, midwives and nursing associates. | | | | | |

## RED FLAGS

Candidate takes the sample from the incorrect port, either leg bag emptying port or water balloon port.

Another Red flag issue (leading directly to patient harm) identified by assessor.

# Notes

# MIDSTREAM SPECIMEN OF URINE (MSU) AND URINALYSIS

| Feedback Score: | Attempt: | 1 | 2 | 3 | 4 | 5 |
|---|---|---|---|---|---|---|
| **Fully Met (2)** **Partially Met (1)** **Not Met (0)** | **Date & Name:** | | | | | |
| 1 | Discusses the procedure with the person and gains consent. | | | | | |
| 2 | Explains to the person how to perform MSU (women to part labia and clean meatus with soap and water from front to back, men to retract foreskin and clean around meatus). Urinate a small amount and then stop flow of urine. Hold the specimen pot a few centimetres away from urethra and urinate until cup is approximately half full. | | | | | |
| 3 | Cleans hands with alcohol hand rub, or washes with soap and water, dries with paper towels, | | | | | |

| | | | | | | |
|---|---|---|---|---|---|---|
| | following WHO guidelines. | | | | | |
| 4 | Checks that all the equipment required for the procedure is available and where applicable, is sterile (i.e., that packaging is undamaged, intact and dry, that sterility indicators are present on any sterilised items and have changed colour where applicable). | | | | | |
| 5 | Gives person clean specimen pot. (Assessor then hands sample to candidate). | | | | | |
| 6 | Dons a disposable plastic apron and non-sterile gloves. | | | | | |
| 7 | Dips reagent strip into the urine for no longer than 1 second. | | | | | |
| 8 | Holds strip at an angle at the edge of the container. | | | | | |
| 9 | Waits the required time before reading the strip against the colour chart - verbalisation accepted. | | | | | |
| 10 | Dispose of equipment appropriately - verbalisation accepted. | | | | | |
| 11 | Cleans hands with alcohol hand rub, or washes with soap and water and dries with paper towels, following WHO guidelines - verbalisation accepted. | | | | | |
| 12 | Identifies the possible significance of the findings, provides appropriate health information to the person according to results, and | | | | | |

| | | | | | | |
|---|---|---|---|---|---|---|
| | informs of actions to be taken next. | | | | | |
| 13 | Accurately documents readings according to reagent strip. | | | | | |
| 14 | Acts professionally throughout the procedure in accordance with NMC (2018) 'The Code: Professional standards of practice and behaviour for nurses, midwives and nursing associates. | | | | | |

## RED FLAGS

Failure to demonstrate ability to read urinalysis strip or record the results accurately correctly should receive a fail.

Another Red flag issue (leading directly to patient harm) identified by assessor.

# <u>Notes</u>

# PEAK EXPIRATORY FLOW RATE (PEFR)

| Feedback Score: | Attempt: | 1 | 2 | 3 | 4 | 5 |
|---|---|---|---|---|---|---|
| **Fully Met (2)** **Partially Met (1)** **Not Met (0)** | **Date & Name:** | | | | | |
| 1 | Explains the procedure to the person and obtains their consent. | | | | | |
| 2 | Cleans hands with alcohol hand rub, or washes with soap and water and dries with paper towels following WHO guidelines. Dons non sterile gloves and apron. | | | | | |
| 3 | Assembles equipment. | | | | | |
| 4 | Asks and assists the person to sit in an upright position. | | | | | |
| 5 | Inserts a disposable mouthpiece into the peak flow meter or uses a single - use/reusable peak flow meter. | | | | | |
| 6 | Ensures that the needle on the gauge is pushed down to zero. | | | | | |
| 7 | Asks the person to hold the peak flow meter horizontally, | | | | | |

| | | | | | | |
|---|---|---|---|---|---|---|
| | ensuring that their fingers do not impede the gauge. | | | | | |
| 8 | Asks the person to take a deep breath in through their mouth to full inspiration. | | | | | |
| 9 | Asks the person to place their lips lightly around the mouthpiece immediately, obtaining a tight seal. | | | | | |
| 10 | Asks the person to blow out through the meter in a short sharp 'huff' as forcefully as they can. | | | | | |
| 11 | Takes a note of the reading and returns the needle on the gauge to zero. Asks the person to take a moment to rest and then to repeat the procedure twice, noting the reading each time. | | | | | |
| 12 | Accurately documents the highest of the three acceptable readings. | | | | | |
| 13 | Disposes of equipment appropriately - verbalisation accepted. | | | | | |
| 14 | Cleans hands with alcohol hand rub, or washes with soap and water and dries with paper towels following WHO guidelines - verbalisation accepted. | | | | | |
| 15 | Acts professionally throughout the procedure in accordance with NMC (2018) 'The Code: Professional standards of practice and behaviour for nurses, midwives and nursing associates. | | | | | |

## RED FLAGS

Candidate is unable to conduct the correct procedure of PEFR, for example advising correct positioning/technique to the patient, or not recording the correct reading.

Another Red Flag issue (leading directly to patient harm) identified by assessor.

# <u>Notes</u>

# ADMINISTRATION OF INHALED MEDICATION (AIM)

| Feedback Score: | Attempt: | 1 | 2 | 3 | 4 | 5 |
|---|---|---|---|---|---|---|
| **Fully Met (2)** **Partially Met (1)** **Not Met (0)** | **Date & Name:** | | | | | |
| 1 | Introduces self, explains procedure and gains consent. | | | | | |
| 2 | Cleans hands with alcohol hand rub, or washes with soap and water and dries with paper towels, following WHO guidelines. | | | | | |
| 3 | Requests/assists the person to sit in an upright position. | | | | | |
| 4 | Before administering any prescribed drug, looks at the person's prescription chart and correctly checks all the following: Correct<br>　　- Person (check ID with person: Verbally, against wristband (Where appropriate) | | | | | |

| | | | | | | |
|---|---|---|---|---|---|---|
| | and documentation)<br>   - drug<br>   - dose<br>   - date and time of administration<br>   - route and method of administration<br>   - diluent (as appropriate)<br>   - Any allergies. | | | | | |
| 5 | Correctly checks all of the following:<br>   - Validity of prescription<br>   - signature of prescriber<br>   - prescription is legible<br>   If any of these pieces of information is missing, unclear or illegible, the nurse should not proceed with administration and should consult the prescriber. | | | | | |
| 6 | Removes the mouthpiece cover from the inhaler. | | | | | |
| 7 | Shakes inhaler well 2 - 5 seconds. | | | | | |
| 8 | With a spacer device: Inserts metered dose inhaler (MDI) into end of spacer device. Asks the person to exhale completely and then to grasp the spacer mouthpiece with their teeth and lips while holding inhaler, ensuring lips form a seal. | | | | | |
| 9 | Asks the person to tip head back slightly, and inhale slowly and deeply through the mouth while depressing the canister fully. | | | | | |
| 10 | Instructs the person in use 'single - breath technique': | | | | | |

| | | | | | | | |
|---|---|---|---|---|---|---|---|
| | breathe in slowly for 2 - 3 seconds and had their breath for approximately 10 seconds, then remove the MDI form mouth before exhaling slowly through pursed lips<br>Or<br>Instructs the person to use 'tidal breathing or 'multi breath technique' if the person can't hold their breath for more than 5 seconds (breathing in and out steadily five minutes). | | | | | | |
| 11 | Ensures the drug is administered as prescribed. | | | | | | |
| 12 | Instructs the person to wait 30 - 60 seconds between inhalations (if same medication) or 2 - 3 minutes between inhalations (if different medication), and shakes the inhaler between doses. | | | | | | |
| 13 | Cleans any equipment used and discards all disposable equipment in appropriate containers. | | | | | | |
| 14 | Cleans hands with alcohol hand rub, or washes with soap and water and dries with paper towels, following WHO guidelines - verbalisation accepted. | | | | | | |
| 15 | Dates and signs drug administration record (prompt permitted) - verbalisation accepted. | | | | | | |
| 16 | Reassures the person appropriately. Closes the | | | | | | |

| | | | | | | | |
|---|---|---|---|---|---|---|---|
| | interaction professionally and appropriately. | | | | | | |
| 17 | Acts professionally throughout the procedure in accordance with NMC (2018) 'The Code: Professional standards of practice and behaviour for nurses, midwives and nursing associates. | | | | | | |

## RED FLAGS

Safety of administration of medication. This should include:

Checking prescription against patient,

Right dose/right time/right patient/right route/right drug.

The chart should then be signed.

If any of this is missed, this should result in a fail.

Another Red flag issue (leading directly to patient harm) identified by assessor.

# <u>Notes</u>

# IN HOSPITAL RESUSCITATION

| Feedback Score: | | Attempt: | 1 | 2 | 3 | 4 | 5 |
|---|---|---|---|---|---|---|---|
| Fully Met (2) Partially Met (1) Not Met (0) | | Date & Name: | | | | | |
| 1 | Ensures personal safety (safe environment). | | | | | | |
| 2 | Checks the person for a response. Shakes shoulders, asks 'Are you alright?' | | | | | | |
| 3 | Shouts for help when the person does not respond (if not done already) | | | | | | |
| 4 | Turns the person onto their back. | | | | | | |
| 5 | Opens airway and looks for any signs of obstruction. | | | | | | |
| 6 | Opens the airway using head tilt and chin lift (jaw - thrust if risk of cervical spine injury). | | | | | | |
| 7 | Establishes absence of breathing normally - for unto 10 seconds.  - looks for chest movement  - listens at the mouth for | | | | | | |

| | | | | | | |
|---|---|---|---|---|---|---|
| | breathing<br>    - Feels for air on their cheek<br>    - checks for carotid pulse<br>(can be done at the same time as listening for breath). | | | | | | |
| 8 | Establishes no signs of life and calls 2222. Ensures resuscitation team are called and resuscitation equipment requested (if alone, leaves the person to get help and equipment). | | | | | | |
| 9 | Starts chest compressions:<br>    - lower half of sternum<br>    - heel of one hand on top of the other<br>    - no pressure on the rib, abdomen and lower sternum<br>    - arms straight | | | | | | |
| 10 | Performs effective chest compressions:<br>    - Compression depth 5 - 6 cm<br>    - Rate 100 - 120 compressions per minute. | | | | | | |
| 11 | After 30 chest compressions, completes 2 ventilations:<br>    - Head tilt<br>    - gives ventilation while watching the chest rise over about1 second (using a bag valve mask)<br>    - pauses, watching for the chest to fall<br>    - gives a second ventilation<br>    - the two ventilations should take no more than 5 seconds | | | | | | |
| 12 | Recommences chest compressions and continues resuscitation with correct | | | | | | |

| | | | | | | | |
|---|---|---|---|---|---|---|---|
| | compression: ventilation ration 30:2. | | | | | | |
| 13 | Acts professionally throughout the procedure in accordance with NMC (2018) 'The Code: Professional standards of practice and behaviour for nurses, midwives and nursing associates. | | | | | | |

## RED FLAGS

An automatic fail shell be applied if: - the candidate does not call for help - the candidate is unable to demonstrate effective cardiopulmonary resuscitation (CPR). This should include inadequate airway support, or ineffective breaths or chest compressions.

# **Notes**

# FLUID BALANCE (FB)

| Feedback Score: | | Attempt: | 1 | 2 | 3 | 4 | 5 |
|---|---|---|---|---|---|---|---|
| **Fully Met (2) Partially Met (1) Not Met (0)** | | **Date & Name:** | | | | | |
| 1 | Hand writing is clear and legible. | | | | | | |
| 2 | Accurately transposes the information onto the fluid balance chart. | | | | | | |
| 3 | Calculates the fluid intake balance accurately. | | | | | | |
| 4 | Calculates the fluid output balance accurately. | | | | | | |
| 5 | Calculates and documents the total fluid balance accurately. | | | | | | |
| 6 | Denotes negative or positive balance accurately. | | | | | | |
| 7 | Ensures strike through errors retains legibility. | | | | | | |
| 8 | Prints and signs name on the chart. | | | | | | |

**RED FLAGS**

Candidate miscalculates the total fluid balance, denoting incorrect negative or positive balance.

Another red flag issue (leading directly to patient harm) identified by assessor.

# <u>Notes</u>

# FINE BORE NG TUBE INSERTION

| Feedback Score: | Attempt: | 1 | 2 | 3 | 4 | 5 |
|---|---|---|---|---|---|---|
| Fully Met (2) Partially Met (1) Not Met (0) | Date & Name: | | | | | |
| 1 | Introduces self | | | | | |
| 2 | Cleans hands with alcohol hand rub, or washes with soap and water and dries with paper towels following WHO guidelines. | | | | | |
| 3 | Assembles the equipment required and dons a disposable plastic apron and non-sterile gloves. | | | | | |
| 4 | Arranges a signal with the patient so that they can communicate if they wish to halt/stop, e.g. raising hand. | | | | | |
| 5 | Assists the patient to sit in a semi upright position in chair/bed, supporting head with pillows to ensure no head tilt forward or backwards. | | | | | |
| 6 | Performs a NEX measurement by measuring the distance | | | | | |

| | | | | | | |
|---|---|---|---|---|---|---|
| | from the patient's nose to their earlobe plus the distance from the earlobe to the bottom of the xiphisternum, adding 5 - 10cm (if candidate does not add 5 - 10 cm, this is not a fail), taking note of the measurement marks on the tube. | | | | | |
| 7 | Checks that the nostrils are patent by asking the patient to sniff with one nostril closed. Repeats with other nostril. | | | | | |
| 8 | Lubricates approx. 15 - 20 cm of the tube with warm water. | | | | | |
| 9 | Ensures a receiver is to hand, in case the patient vomits. Ensure there is working oxygen and suction at the bedside. | | | | | |
| 10 | Inserts proximal end of the tube into the nostril, and slides backwards and inwards along the floor of the nose to the nasopharynx. Stops if encounters any obstruction and tries again in a a slightly different direction or uses other nostril. | | | | | |
| 11 | Asks the patient to start swallowing if they are able to, as tube passes down nasopharynx into the oesophagus. | | | | | |
| 12 | Advances the tube through the pharynx as patient swallows until the measured indicator on the tube reaches the entrance of the nostril. | | | | | |
| 13 | Recognises any signs of distress such as coughing or breathlessness, when the tube would should be removed | | | | | |

| | | | | | | | |
|---|---|---|---|---|---|---|---|
| | immediately. | | | | | | |
| 14 | Uses adherent dressing tape to secure the tube to nostril and cheek. | | | | | | |
| 15 | Aspirates a small amount of the stomach contents using a 50 ml or 60 ml syringe, confirming that the tube is in position by using a pH indicator strip to confirm the presence of acid (the pH should be equal to or less than 5.5). Uses integral cap to cap the tube. | | | | | | |
| 16 | Disposes of equipment including apron and gloves appropriately - verbalisation accepted. | | | | | | |
| 17 | Cleans hands with alcohol hand rub or washes with soap and water and dries with paper towels following WHO guidelines - verbalisation accepted. | | | | | | |
| 18 | Ensures that the patient is comfortable post procedure. | | | | | | |
| 19 | States the additional checks that may be undertaken to check tube positioning before commencing feeding (i.e., further checking with pH indicator strip immediately prior to each feed/ in very specific circumstances radiologically). | | | | | | |
| 20 | Acts professionally throughout the procedure in accordance with NMC (2018)'The Code: Professional standards of practice and behaviour for nurses, midwives and nursing associates. | | | | | | |

## RED FLAGS

Candidate does not recognise the significance of displaced tube, i.e., is not able to state what the pH should be to confirm the correct tube positioning.

Candidates does not recognise the significance of additional she checks prior to commencing feeding.

Another Red Flag issue (leading directly to patient harm) identified by assessor.

# **<u>Notes</u>**

# INTRA-VENOUS FLUSH AND VIP SCORING

| Feedback Score: | Attempt: | 1 | 2 | 3 | 4 | 5 |
|---|---|---|---|---|---|---|
| Fully Met (2) Partially Met (1) Not Met (0) | Date & Name: | | | | | |
| 1 | Checks that all the equipment required for the procedure is available and, where applicable, is sterile (i.e., that packaging is undamaged, intact and dry, that sterility indicators are present on any sterilised items and have changed colour, where applicable). | | | | | |
| 2 | Assesses the cannula and verbalises signs of phlebitis pain, erythema (colour), oedema, palpable venous cord, pyrexia (identifies two for a partial and five for a full pass). | | | | | |
| 3 | Cleans hands with alcohol hand rub, or washes with soap and water and dries with paper towels, following WHO guidelines. | | | | | |

| | | | | | | |
|---|---|---|---|---|---|---|
| 4 | States that the tray or trolley has been cleaned with detergent wipes (or equivalent) and places all the equipment required for the procedure on the bottom shelf of the clean dressing trolley (or suitable equivalent). | | | | | |
| 5 | Dons a disposable plastic apron. | | | | | |
| 6 | Takes the equipment to the person's bedside in tray or trolley. | | | | | |
| 7 | Gains consent and explains the procedure to the patient. | | | | | |
| 8 | Before administering any prescribed drugs, looks at the persons prescription chart and correctly checks all of the following: Correct:     - Person (checks ID with person: verbally, against wristband (where appropriate) and documentation).     - drug     - dose     - date and time of administration     - route and method of administration     - diluent (as appropriate)     - any allergies | | | | | |
| 9 | Correctly checks all of the following:     - Validity of prescription     - Signature of prescriber     - prescription is legible. If any of these pieces of information is missing, unclear or illegible, the nurse should not proceed with administration | | | | | |

| | | | | | | |
|---|---|---|---|---|---|---|
| | and should consult the prescriber. | | | | | |
| 10 | Cleans hands with alcohol hand rub, or washes with soap and water and dries with paper towels. Dons non sterile gloves. | | | | | |
| 11 | Cleanses the end of the IV port with sterile alcohol wipes saturated with 70% isopropyl alcohol for 30 seconds, leaving to dry over 30 seconds. | | | | | |
| 12 | Connects the pre filled syringe to the port using an aseptic non touch technique (ANTT) and flushes cannula using a pulsating action. | | | | | |
| 13 | Asks the patient whether any discomfort is experienced while flushing. | | | | | |
| 14 | Disposes of waste appropriately - verbalisation accepted. | | | | | |
| 15 | Cleans hands with alcohol hand rub, or washes with soap and water and dries with paper towels, following WHO guidelines - verbalisation accepted. | | | | | |
| 16 | Dates and signs drug administration record. Prompt permitted - verbalisation accepted. | | | | | |
| 17 | Acts professionally throughout the procedure in accordance with NMC (2018)'The Code: Professional standards of practice and behaviour for nurses, midwives and nursing associates. | | | | | |

## RED FLAGS

If the candidate fails to administer the medication correctly.
They must check the following:
- Right patient/dose/time/route/drug.
- They must also sign, date and time the prescription.
- If any of the above is missed, this should result in a fail

If candidate does not use aseptic non touch technique for the procedure/contaminates the sterile areas, this should result in a fail.

Another Red Flag issue (leading directly to patient harm) identified by assessor.

# <u>Notes</u>

# PRESSURE AREA ASSESSMENT

| Feedback Score: | Attempt: | 1 | 2 | 3 | 4 | 5 |
|---|---|---|---|---|---|---|
| **Fully Met (2) Partially Met (1) Not Met (0)** | **Date & Name:** | | | | | |
| 1 | Identifies the most vulnerable areas of pressure risk. Either formal anatomical or plain English can be used.<br>• Heels<br>• Sacrum<br>• Ischial tuberosities (buttocks)<br>• Elbows<br>• Temporal region of the skull<br>• Shoulders<br>• Femoral trochanters (hips)<br>• Back of head<br>• Toes<br>• Ears<br>• Spine<br><br>8 Areas need to be identified for full marks and 5 areas for partial marks | | | | | |
| 2 | Identifies signs that may indicate pressure ulcer development: | | | | | |

| | | | | | | |
|---|---|---|---|---|---|---|
| | • Persistent erythema (flushing of the skin)<br>• Non blanching hyperaemia (discolouration of the skin that does not change when pressed).<br>• Blisters<br>• Discolouration<br>• Localised heat<br>• Localised oedema<br>• Localised indurations (abnormal hardening)<br>• Purplish/bluish localised areas<br>• Localised coolness if tissue death has occurred<br><br>7 areas need to be identified for full marks and 4 areas for partial marks | | | | | |
| 3 | Completes the Braden tool accurately, and correctly calculates the sub scores and overall score based on the patient scenario and pressure damage identified. | | | | | |
| 4 | Documents findings accurately, clearly and legibly. | | | | | |

## RED FLAGS

Failure to recognise damage OR miscalculates the score, resulting in no action. Either of these should result in a fail for this station.

Another red flag issue (leading directly to patient harm) identified by assessor.

# Notes

# BLOOD GLUCOSE MONITORING

| Feedback Score: | Attempt: | 1 | 2 | 3 | 4 | 5 |
|---|---|---|---|---|---|---|
| **Fully Met (2)** **Partially Met (1)** **Not Met (0)** | **Date & Name:** | | | | | |
| 1 | Assembles the equipment required and checks that the strips are in date and have not been exposed to air. | | | | | |
| 2 | Explains the procedure with the person, gains consent. | | | | | |
| 3 | Cleans own hand with alcohol hand rub, or washes with soap and water and dries with paper towels, following WHO guidelines. | | | | | |
| 4 | Dons a disposable plastic apron and non-sterile gloves. | | | | | |
| 5 | Checks that the patient's hands are visibly clean. | | | | | |
| 6 | Takes a single use lancet and takes blood sample from the side of finger, ensuring that the site of piercing is rotated. Avoids use of index finger and thumb. | | | | | |

| 7 | Inserts the testing strip into the glucometer and applies blood to the strip. Ensures that the window on the test strip is entirely covered with blood. | | | | | |
|---|---|---|---|---|---|---|
| 8 | Gives the patient a piece of gauze to stop the bleeding. | | | | | |
| 9 | Ensures that all sharps and non-sharp waste are disposed of safely (including scooping method of re 0 sheathing, if used and transportation of sharps) and in accordance with locally approved procedures. | | | | | |
| 10 | Cleans hands with alcohol hand rub, or washes with soap and water and dries with paper towels, following WHO guidelines - Verbalisation accepted. | | | | | |
| 11 | Verbalises whether the result is within normal limits and indicates whether any action is required. | | | | | |
| 12 | Documents the result accurately, clearly and legibly. | | | | | |
| 13 | Acts professionally throughout the procedure in accordance with NMC (2018) 'The Code: Professional standards of practice and behaviour for nurses, midwives and nursing associates. | | | | | |

## **RED FLAGS**

Candidate does not demonstrate knowledge of normal range of blood glucose or does not act appropriately/acknowledge abnormal reading.

Another Red Flag issue (leading directly to patient harm) identified by assessor.

# <u>Notes</u>

# PAIN ASSESSMENT

| Feedback Score: | Attempt: | 1 | 2 | 3 | 4 | 5 |
|---|---|---|---|---|---|---|
| Fully Met (2) Partially Met (1) Not Met (0) | Date & Name: | | | | | |
| 1 | Introduces self and explains the assessment to be carried out and the rationale and importance of this. | | | | | |
| 2 | Gains consent from the patient. Identifies the patient by checking name/date of birth or ID. | | | | | |
| 3 | Considers the following aspects of pain | | | | | |
| 3a | P = provokes Where is the pain? (Point to area) What causes the pain? What makes it better? What makes it worse? | | | | | |
| 3b | Q = quality What does the pain feel like? Is it dull, sharp, stabbing, burning, crushing, shooting, throbbing? Is the pain intense? | | | | | |
| 3c | R = radiating Where is it? Is it in one place? Does it move around? | | | | | |

| | | | | | | | |
|---|---|---|---|---|---|---|---|
| | Did is start somewhere else? | | | | | | |
| 3d | S = severity How bad is it? Uses the universal pain scale to ascertain severity. | | | | | | |
| 3e | T = time When did the pain start? How long has it lasted? Is to constant? Does it come and go? Is it sudden or gradual? | | | | | | |
| 4 | Acknowledges that the patient is in discomfort, and offers to make them more comfortable by repositioning. | | | | | | |
| 5 | Asks patient whether they have had any analgesia, and states will arrange for suitable analgesia. | | | | | | |
| 6 | Identifies the need to communicate with multidisciplinary team/doctor. | | | | | | |
| 7 | Identifies the need for regular reassessment. | | | | | | |
| 8 | Indicates the need to document findings accurately and clearly in the patient notes/charts. | | | | | | |
| 9 | Reassures the patient. | | | | | | |
| 10 | Acts professionally throughout the procedure in accordance with NMC (2018) 'The Code: Professional standards of practice and behaviour for nurses, midwives and nursing associates. | | | | | | |

## RED FLAGS

Any Red flag issue (leading directly to patient harm) identified by assessor.

# **Notes**

# ADMINISTRATION OF SUPPOSITORY

| Feedback Score: | Attempt: | 1 | 2 | 3 | 4 | 5 |
|---|---|---|---|---|---|---|
| **Fully Met (2)** **Partially Met (1)** **Not Met (0)** | **Date & Name:** | | | | | |
| 1 | Introduces self, explains procedure and gains consent. | | | | | |
| 2 | Cleans hands with alcohol hand rub, or washes with soap and water and dries with paper towels following WHO guidelines. | | | | | |
| 3 | Assembles the equipment required (Bedpan, commode or toilet) and dons a plastic apron and non-sterile gloves. | | | | | |
| 4 | Verbalises that they would request/assist the person to lie on their left lateral side with knees flexed, fleet level or slightly raised, buttocks near to the edge of the bed (the manikin should not be moved into position for health and safety reasons). | | | | | |

| | | | | | | |
|---|---|---|---|---|---|---|
| 5 | Places a disposable incontinence pad beneath the patient's hips and buttocks. | | | | | |
| 6 | Before administering any prescribed drug, looks at the person's prescription chart and checks that All of the following are correct:<br>• person (checks id with person: verbally, against wristband (where appropriate) and documentation)<br>• Drug<br>• Dose<br>• Date and time of administration<br>• Route and method of administration<br>• Diluent (as appropriate)<br>• Any allergies | | | | | |
| 7 | Correctly checks All of the following<br>• Validity of prescription<br>• Signature of prescriber<br>• Prescription is legible<br>If any of these pieces of information is missing, unclear or illegible, the nurse should not proceed with administration and should consult the prescriber. | | | | | |
| 8 | Prior to inserting the suppository, verbalises that they are observing the anal area for evidence of skin soreness, excoriation, swelling, haemorrhoids, rectal prolapse or infestation. | | | | | |
| 9 | Place some lubricating jelly on | | | | | |

| | | | | | | |
|---|---|---|---|---|---|---|
| | a gauze square and lubricates the suppository. Separates the patient's buttocks and inserts the suppository using the correct end (referring to the manufactures instructions), advancing it approximately 2 cm to 4 cm. Repeats this procedure if additional suppositories are to be inserted. | | | | | |
| 10 | Cleans any excess lubricating jelly from the patient's perineal and perianal areas using gauze squares after insertion of suppository. | | | | | |
| 11 | Verbalises that they would advise the patient to remain lying down and retain the suppository for about 20 minutes or until they are no longer able to do so. Informs the patient that there may be some discharge as the medication melts int the rectum. | | | | | |
| 12 | Verbalises that they would assists the patient into a comfortable position and offers a bedpan, commode or toilet facility, as appropriate. | | | | | |
| 13 | Maintains patient dignity: arranges the bedcovers to keep the patient covered as much as possible during the procedure and replaces patient's bedclothes and covers once the suppository has been inserted. | | | | | |
| 14 | Disposes of waste appropriately and cleans any equipment used. | | | | | |
| 15 | Cleans hands with alcohol | | | | | |

| | | | | | | |
|---|---|---|---|---|---|---|
| | hand rub, or washes with soap and water, and dries with paper towels following WHO guidelines - verbalisation accepted. | | | | | |
| 16 | Dates and signs medicines administration record. | | | | | |
| 17 | Reassures the person appropriately. Closes the interaction professionally and appropriately. | | | | | |
| 18 | Acts professionally throughout the procedure in accordance with NMC (2018) 'The Code: Professional standards of practice and behaviour for nurses, midwives and nursing associates. | | | | | |

## **RED FLAGS**

Safety of administration of medication. This should include:

Checking prescription against patient.

Right dose/right time/ right patient/right route/right drug.

The chart should then be signed.

If any of this is missed, this should result in a fail.

Another red flag issue (leading directly to patient harm) identified by assessor.

# <u>Notes</u>

# BOWEL ASSESSMENT

| Feedback Score: | | Attempt: | 1 | 2 | 3 | 4 | 5 |
|---|---|---|---|---|---|---|---|
| **Fully Met (2)** **Partially Met (1)** **Not Met (0)** | | **Date & Name:** | | | | | |
| 1 | Completes the Bristol stool chart accurately, and signs, dates and adds time where required. | | | | | | |
| 2 | Handwriting is clear and legible. | | | | | | |
| 3 | Ensures that strike through errors retains legibility. | | | | | | |
| 4a | If using photo, **A or B:**<br>• Correctly recognises Bristol stool type 1 or 2 appropriately and proposes plan of care to reduce/prevent constipation:<br>• Considers possible causes of constipation, such as medication and explores potential alternatives.<br>• Offers dietary advice (increasing fibre, fruit and vegetables)<br>• Proposes obtaining a prescription for laxatives<br>• Considers dehydration and encourages increased fluid intake. | | | | | | |

| | | | | | | | |
|---|---|---|---|---|---|---|---|
| | • Encourages physical movement where possible<br>• Encourages not to ignore the urge to defecate<br>• Promotes positive toilet habits: privacy, positioning, breathing exercises and spending time going to the toilet<br>• Recognises the need to continue to assess bowels<br><br>To achieve full marks, the candidate needs to identify a minimum of five aspects of care.<br><br>For partial marks, the candidate needs to identify a minimum of three aspects of care. | | | | | | |
| 4b | If using photo **C or D**:<br>• Correctly recognises Bristol stool type 6 or 7 appropriately and proposes plan of care to reduce/prevent diarrhoea:<br>• Considers possible causes of loose stool: food poisoning, overflow, medication such as antibiotics, healthcare acquired infection such as norovirus or Clostridium difficile, or malabsorption.<br>• Considers infection - control measures: patient isolation, sending sample for culture<br>• Offer dietary advice (reducing fruit and vegetables)<br>• Proposes obtaining a prescription of anti-motility medication if suspected non-infectious cause. | | | | | | |

| | | | | | | |
|---|---|---|---|---|---|---|
| | • Considers dehydration and encourages increased fluid intake.<br>• Considers perianal skin integrity.<br>• Promotes positive toilet habits: privacy, positioning, close proximity to toilet/ commode and spending time going to the toilet.<br>• Recognises the need to continue to assess bowels.<br><br>To achieve full marks, the candidate needs to identify a minimum of five aspects of care. | | | | | |
| 5 | Acts professionally throughout the procedure in accordance with NMC (2018) 'The Code: Professional standards of practice and behaviour for nurses, midwives and nursing associates. | | | | | |

## RED FLAGS

Candidate does not complete the Bristol stool chart accurately. (Inappropriate identification of stool type)

Another Red flag issue (leading Directly to patient harm) identified by assessor.

# <u>Notes</u>

# NASOPHARYNGEAL SUCTIONING

| Feedback Score: | Attempt: | 1 | 2 | 3 | 4 | 5 |
|---|---|---|---|---|---|---|
| **Fully Met (2) Partially Met (1) Not Met (0)** | **Date & Name:** | | | | | |
| 1 | Cleans hands with alcohol hand rub, or washes with soap and water and dries with paper towels, following WHO guidelines. | | | | | |
| 2 | Introduces self. Explains the procedure to be carried out and the rationale for this. | | | | | |
| 3 | Arranges a signal with the patient so that they can communicate if they wish to halt/stop. E.g., Raising hand. | | | | | |
| 4 | States that they will monitor the patient's condition throughout the intervention, i.e., colour, breathing pattern, respiratory rate, heart rate, secretions, and evidence of trauma and distress, using pre suction baseline observations as a guideline. | | | | | |

| 5 | Assists the patient to sit in a semi upright position in chair/ bed, supporting head with pillows and ensuring no head tilt forwards or backwards. | | | | | |
| 6 | Dons a disposable plastic apron, non-sterile gloves, mask and goggles. | | | | | |
| 7 | Checks that the nostrils are patient by asking the patient to sniff with one nostril closed. Repeats with the other nostril. | | | | | |
| 8 | Selects an appropriate type and size of catheter for the task and size of the patient (size 10 or 12 accepted). | | | | | |
| 9 | Sets suction to 12 - 20 kPa/100 - 150 mmHg, and checks suction is working. | | | | | |
| 10 | Assembles equipment using non touch technique, and attaches tubing to the wall suction canister and suction catheter to the tubing. | | | | | |
| 11 | Lubricates the tip of the catheter with sterile water and gently inserts the catheter into the nostril as the patient inhales until the patient coughs or resistance is felt. | | | | | |
| 12 | States that if resistance is felt or distressed caused, such as uncontrolled coughing, the catheter will be withdrawn 1cm before applying suction. | | | | | |
| 13 | Applies suction by placing thumb over valve. Slowly | | | | | |

| | | | | | | | |
|---|---|---|---|---|---|---|---|
| | withdraws, maintaining the vacuum, applying intermittent suctioning (10 second intervals). Rotating, the catheter is withdrawn to avoid damaging structures. States that they would repeat the procedure 2 to 3 times as required/tolerated. | | | | | | |
| 14 | Flushes the suction tubing with sterile water. | | | | | | |
| 15 | Ensures that the patient's face is clean and that they are safe and comfortable post procedure. | | | | | | |
| 16 | Disposes of equipment, including apron and gloves, appropriately - Verbalisation accepted. | | | | | | |
| 17 | Cleans hands with alcohol hand rub, or washes with soap and water and dries with paper towels, following WHO guidelines - verbalisation accepted. | | | | | | |
| 18 | Acts professionally throughout the procedure in accordance with NMC (2018) 'The Code: Professional standards of practice and behaviour for nurses, midwives and nursing associates. | | | | | | |

## RED FLAGS

Candidate does not demonstrate appropriate suctioning technique. If any of this is missed, this should result in a fail.

Another Red flag issue (leading Directly to patient harm) identified by assessor.

# <u>Notes</u>

# NUTRITIONAL ASSESSMENT

| Feedback Score: | | Attempt: | 1 | 2 | 3 | 4 | 5 |
|---|---|---|---|---|---|---|---|
| Fully Met (2) Partially Met (1) Not Met (0) | | Date & Name: | | | | | |
| 1 | Accurately calculates the BMI and the score in step 1 of the malnutrition universal screening tool (MUST). | | | | | | |
| 2 | Identifies the percentage of weight loss and accurately calculates the score in step 2 of MUST. | | | | | | |
| 3 | Interprets the clinical information provided and accurately calculates the score in step 3 of MUST. | | | | | | |
| 4 | Accurately calculates an overall risk score and identifies the correct risk category. | | | | | | |
| 5 | Documents date, time and signature where required. | | | | | | |
| 6 | Verbally reports the findings to the examiner. | | | | | | |

| 7 | Verbally recognises that the patient will need referring to a dietician or nutritional support team. | | | | | |
|---|---|---|---|---|---|---|
| 8 | Verbally proposes a plan to improve nutritional intake. | | | | | |
| 9 | Verbally proposes monitoring the patient's nutritional status. | | | | | |
| 10 | Verbally considers possible underlying causes, provides food choices and offers assistance with feeding, if required. | | | | | |
| 11 | Handwriting is clear and legible. | | | | | |
| 12 | Ensures that strike through errors retain legibility. | | | | | |
| 13 | Acts professionally throughout the procedure in accordance with NMC (2018) 'The Code: Professional standards of practice and behaviour for nurses, midwives and nursing associates. | | | | | |

## RED FLAGS

Candidate does not calculate MUST score correctly.
Another Red Flag issue (leading directly to patient harm) identified by assessor.

# **<u>Notes</u>**

# ORAL CARE PLAN

| Feedback Score: | Attempt: | 1 | 2 | 3 | 4 | 5 |
|---|---|---|---|---|---|---|
| **Fully Met (2) Partially Met (1) Not Met (0)** | **Date & Name:** | | | | | |
| 1 | Handwriting is clear and legible. | | | | | |
| 2 | Ensures that strike through errors retain legibility | | | | | |
| 3 | Recommends specific action to be taken depending on scenario. | | | | | |
| 3a | **Cerys Jones (Critical Care) scenario**<br>• Twice daily teeth cleaning with soft, compact headed toothbrush or a suction toothbrush.<br>• Twice daily chlorhexidine mouthwash to reduce the risk of ventilator associated pneumonia.<br>• Apply oral moisturiser to the oral mucosa and lip balm to the lips every 2 to 4 hours.<br>• Minimise traumatic ulceration caused by endotracheal tubes by using specifically designed fasteners | | | | | |

| | | | | | | |
|---|---|---|---|---|---|---|
| | and bite block, and alternating tubing from side to side<br>• Use suction to prevent aspiration, as required<br>• Identifies the need for regular reassessment every 8 hours.<br>• Or/and the candidate identifies an aspect of care that is relevant and evidence based in addition to the list above.<br><br>To achieve full marks, the candidate needs to identify a minimum of six aspects of care.<br><br>For partial marks, the candidate needs to identify a minimum of three aspects of care. | | | | | | |
| 3b | **Luca Saunders (learning and physical disability) scenario**<br>• Twice - daily teeth cleaning with soft, compact - headed toothbrush or electric toothbrush.<br>• Encourage self-care, using a foam handle to assist with holding a toothbrush and pump action toothpaste.<br>• Regular oral mouth cleansing/swabbing/hydration (ice chips or sips of water) throughout the day.<br>• Mouthwash if able to tolerate.<br>• Keeps lips clean and moist using moisturiser/lip balm.<br>• Regular wiping of face to minimise moisture on skin and use of moisturising barrier cream on lower jaw to protect | | | | | | |

| | | | | | | | |
|---|---|---|---|---|---|---|---|
| | skin from drool.<br>• Or/and the candidate identifies an aspect of care that is relevant and evidence based in addition to the list above.<br><br>To achieve full marks, the candidate needs to identify a minimum of six aspects of care.<br><br>For partial marks, the candidate needs to identify a minimum of three aspects of care. | | | | | | |
| 3c | **Michael Watts (cancer treatment) scenario**<br><br>• Twice daily teeth cleaning with soft toothbrush, if able to tolerate.<br>• Twice daily chlorhexidine mouthwash, if able to tolerate.<br>• Regular oral cleansing/ hydration (ice chips or sips of water) throughout the day.<br>• Apply oral moisturiser to the oral mucosa and lip balm to the lips every 2 to 4 hours.<br>• Use of artificial saliva.<br>• Offers analgesia.<br>• Identifies the need for 8 hourly reassessments.<br>• Or/and the candidate identifies an aspect of care that is relevant and evidence based in addition to the list above.<br>To achieve full marks, the candidate needs to identify a minimum of six aspects of care.<br>For partial marks, the candidate needs to identify a minimum of three aspects of care. | | | | | | |

| | | | | | | |
|---|---|---|---|---|---|---|
| 3d | **Rachel Cohen (end of life) scenario**<br>• Twice daily teeth and denture cleaning with soft toothbrush, if able to tolerate.<br>• Twice daily chlorhexidine mouthwash, if able to tolerate.<br>• Regular oral cleansing and hydration (using spray or dropper or ice chips or sips of water) throughout the day.<br>• Remove dentures overnight and soak them in cleaning solution.<br>• Keep lips clean and moist using moisturiser/lip balm (but not petroleum jelly/Vaseline as on oxygen).<br>• Identifies the need for 8 hourly reassessments.<br>• Or/and the candidate identifies an aspect of care that is relevant and evidence based in addition to the list above.<br>To achieve full marks, the candidate needs to identify a minimum of six aspects of care. For partial marks, the candidate needs to identify a minimum of three aspects of care | | | | | | |
| 4 | Acts professionally throughout the procedure in accordance with NMC (2018) 'The Code: Professional standards of practice and behaviour for nurses, midwives and nursing associates. | | | | | | |

## RED FLAGS

Candidate fails to identifying aspect of care

If any of this is missed, this should result in a fail.

Another Red flag issue (leading Directly to patient harm) identified by assessor.

# **Notes**

# OXYGEN THERAPY

| Feedback Score: | Attempt: | 1 | 2 | 3 | 4 | 5 |
|---|---|---|---|---|---|---|
| **Fully Met (2) Partially Met (1) Not Met (0)** | **Date & Name:** | | | | | |
| 1 | Explains the procedure to the person and discusses it with them. | | | | | |
| 2 | Before administering any prescribed drug, looks at person's prescription chart and checks that all of the following are correct:<br>• Person (Checks ID with person: verbally, against wristband (where appropriate) and documentation)<br>• Target saturations<br>• Device and flow rate<br>• Date and time of administration<br>• Any allergies | | | | | |
| 3 | Correctly checks all of the following:<br>• validity of prescription<br>• Signature of prescriber<br>• Prescription is legible<br>If any of these pieces of | | | | | |

| | | | | | | |
|---|---|---|---|---|---|---|
| | information is missing, unclear or illegible, the nurse should not proceed with administration and should consult the prescriber. | | | | | |
| 4 | Cleans hands with alcohol hand rub, or washes with soap and water and dries with paper towels, following WHO guidelines. | | | | | |
| 5 | Identifies/selects the correct equipment (reservoir mask) and assembles and attaches tubing to the flow meter. | | | | | |
| 6 | Turns the oxygen flow meter on, selecting the correct flow rate of oxygen for the method of delivery (1.5 litres per minute) | | | | | |
| 7 | Covers the one way valve with fingers until the reservoir bag is fully inflated. | | | | | |
| 8 | Applies the oxygen mask by placing over the patient's nose and mouth, then pulls the elastic strap over the head and adjusts the nose brace and straps on both sides to secure the mask in a position that seals the face but is not too tight. | | | | | |
| 9 | Ensures that the chosen delivery method is comfortable for the patient. | | | | | |
| 10 | State that they will reassess the saturations to check whether they are within the normal target range for the patient (94 - 98%), escalating if this is not achieved. | | | | | |

| 11 | States that they will inspect the patient's skin regularly around the face, ears and back of head, and provide regular mouth care. | | | | | |
|----|---|---|---|---|---|---|
| 12 | Signs and dates the drug administration record. | | | | | |
| 13 | Acts professionally throughout the procedure in accordance with NMC (2018) 'The Code: Professional standards of practice and behaviour for nurses, midwives and nursing associates. | | | | | |

## RED FLAGS

Candidate fails to recognise the appropriate delivery device. Instances of hyperventilation or hypoventilation.

If any of this is missed, this should result in a fail.

Another Red Flag issue (leading Directly to patient harm) identified by assessor.

# **<u>Notes</u>**